Hemorrhoids

Hemorrhoid Treatment

Hemorrhoid Prevention

By Ace McCloud
Copyright © 2013

Disclaimer

The information provided in this book is designed to provide helpful information on the subjects discussed. This book is not meant to be used, nor should it be used, to diagnose or treat any medical condition. For diagnosis or treatment of any medical problem, consult your own physician. The publisher and author are not responsible for any specific health or allergy needs that may require medical supervision and are not liable for any damages or negative consequences from any treatment, action, application or preparation, to any person reading or following the information in this book. Any references included are provided for informational purposes only. Readers should be aware that any websites or links listed in this book may change.

Table of Contents

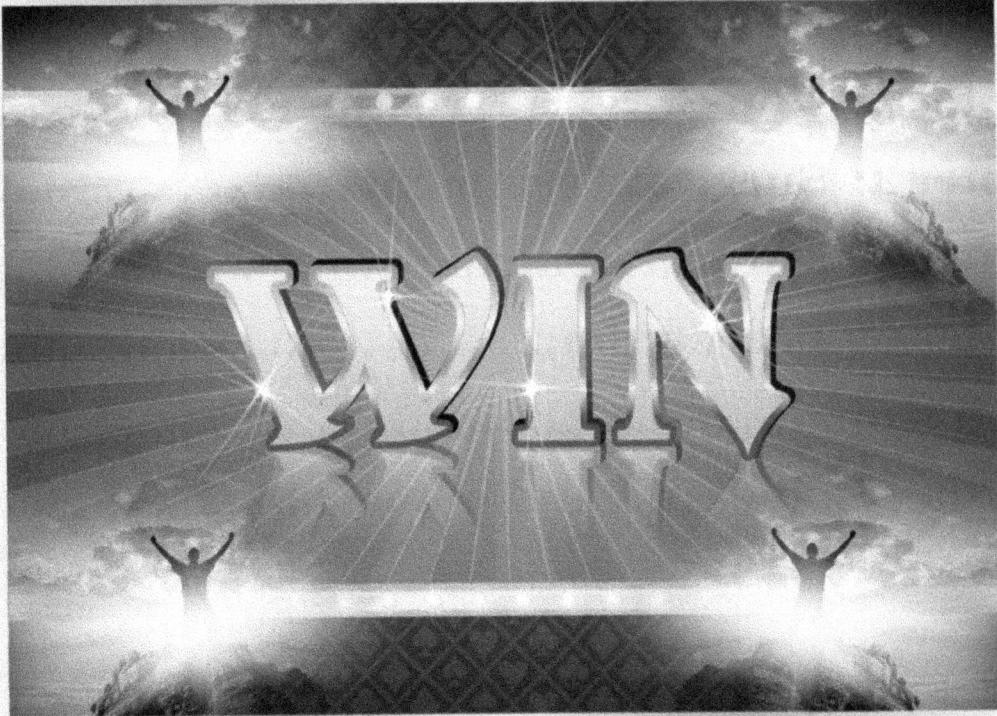

DEDICATED TO THOSE WHO ARE PLAYING THE GAME OF LIFE TO

WIN

KEEP ON PUSHING AND NEVER GIVE UP!

Ace McCloud

Be sure to check out my website for all my Books and Audio books.

www.AcesEbooks.com

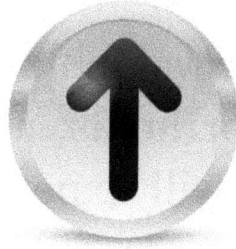

Introduction

I want to thank you and congratulate you for buying the book, 'Hemorrhoid Treatment and Prevention: How To Treat Hemorrhoids And Help Prevent Hemorrhoids From Coming Back.'

This book contains very valuable information on how to treat and prevent hemorrhoids, a condition which about half of the population will experience at some point in their lives. While hemorrhoids rarely evolves into a serious medical issue requiring emergency surgery, both internal and external hemorrhoids can decrease a person's quality of life significantly. Those who suffer from it can experience physical discomfort in the form of intense itchiness and burning sensations around and inside the anal area, along with feelings of embarrassment and worry caused by rectal bleeding during bowel movements. Since the exact cause of hemorrhoids is still a mystery, the medical community agrees that the best way to deal with hemorrhoids is by living a healthy, stress-free lifestyle, which will minimize the chances of suffering from the condition in the first place. This book will offer several suggestions that readers can use to both treat and prevent hemorrhoids from becoming a long-term issue affecting their quality of life.

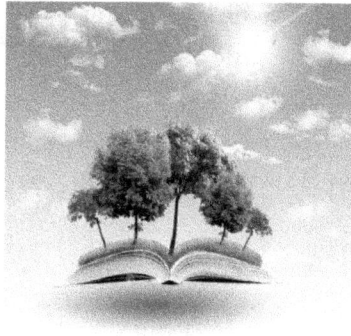

Chapter 1: Overview of Hemorrhoids

The medical condition known as 'hemorrhoids' (also referred to as 'piles') has been causing humans discomfort for thousands of years. The first known mention of it seems to come from an ancient Egyptian papyrus offering healing advice, dating approximately 1700 BC. It states, ". . . Thou shouldest give a recipe, an ointment of great protection; Acacia leaves, ground, titurated and cooked together. Smear a strip of fine linen there-with and place in the anus, that he recovers immediately."

During bowel movements, stool is assisted in exiting the anus by vascular bodies called hemorrhoids. When these structures become inflamed, they can lead to extreme discomfort, both during and after the stool is passed.

Since many people who suffer from the condition do not seek medical treatment, either because of a lack of health insurance, an unwillingness to pay out of pocket expenses, strong feelings of embarrassment, or simply disinterest or laziness, it is difficult to know exactly how many cases of hemorrhoids there are. But the medical community estimates that around half of the US population will at some point in their lives suffer from hemorrhoids, whether it be a mild case or an extreme one.

The percentage of afflicted people tends to be higher among whites compared with other racial and ethnic groups. Age-wise, the highest rates of people suffering from hemorrhoids seem to fall into the forty-five to sixty-five years old demographic. Some famous people who have suffered from hemorrhoids include George Brett and Glenn Beck.

Brett was a star baseball player for the Kansas City Royals who had to be taken out of a 1980 World Series game because he could not tolerate the pain from his hemorrhoids. After receiving medical treatment in the form of very minor surgery, he was able to return for the next game. He remained very good-natured throughout the incident, jokingly telling the press, ". . . my problems are all behind me." Glenn Beck, a popular conservative talk show host, also had to have surgery to deal with his hemorrhoids. While he experienced a complete recovery, he did not pass up the opportunity to criticize the American health care industry, posting a humorous YouTube video that has garnered almost one million views.

Thankfully, hemorrhoids are rarely a life-threatening condition, though in a few cases enough blood loss can occur where the patient can develop anemia (a severe decrease in the number of red blood cells in the body). Hemorrhoids can, however, become a systematically recurring problem for some individuals, but with proper treatment and prevention the disorder will usually heal enough not to cause long-term problems or discomfort.

Chapter 2: Hemorrhoids Defined

Hemorrhoids fall into one of two categories: internal and external, depending on where the enlarged blood vessels lie in the anal cavity. While rarely life-threatening, both kinds of hemorrhoids can cause extreme levels of discomfort and worry for those who suffer from them.

External hemorrhoids lie within the anus, but can enlarge to the point where they can be seen outside of it. When a blood clot forms inside of a blood vessel that obstructs the flow of blood through the circulatory system, it is known as thrombosis. If a patient experiences external hemorrhoids that are not obstructing the flow of blood, they may get away with few, if any problems. If, however, blood clotting is present, the situation can become very painful, as the area can become extremely inflamed and irritated, and can lead to extreme bouts of itchiness in the rectal area that can become worse with each successive bowel movement. Regardless, the pain normally disappears in two to three days time. Unfortunately, it may be a few weeks before the swelling fully goes away. Even after the swelling is gone and the area has healed itself, a skin tag (harmless skin growths that have the appearance of small soft balloons) may remain.

People that experience internal hemorrhoids normally do not feel much in the way of pain (unless blood clotting is also present), and since the inflamed area is far inside the rectum (which contains few pain nerves), it is hard to detect any noticeable symptoms. Bowel movements, however, may be accompanied by various amounts of bleeding. Bleeding during bowel movements can be a source of extreme worry, which is why many people do not seek medical treatment until their hemorrhoids have reached a very advanced stage. Other symptoms of internal hemorrhoids can include small or large amounts of mucous discharge, a mass of tissue protruding from the anus, extreme itchiness, and some loss of control over bowel functions resulting in unexpected defecation. If the hemorrhoids protrude outside the anus, they will appear as a soft, pink mass that can gently be pushed back in over time or removed, as described later in this book.

Doctors are still not clear on what exactly causes hemorrhoids, but several factors are believed to play a role. These include irregular bowel habits, a chronic cough, high frequency of constipation and/or diarrhea, lack of exercise, obesity, poor diet (such as diets low on fiber and nutrition), increased abdominal pressure (due to prolonged straining, lifting, pregnancy, etc.), genetics, prolonged sitting, a lack of functioning valves within the hemorrhoid's veins, and aging. Unfortunately, pregnant women will experience many of the discomforts associated with hemorrhoids, but will rarely require surgical treatment, as symptoms usually clear up on their own after the birth of the child.

Chapter 3: Non-Surgical Treatments

While surgery is usually required to treat serious hemorrhoids, it is not recommended for minor cases. Instead, hemorrhoids can be treated in a doctor's office, or in the privacy of your own home, with various sorts of remedies.

Increasing fiber intake, either through the consumption of natural foods high in fiber or through fiber supplements is highly recommended. It can help ease constipation and eliminate straining during bowel movements, making it less likely for the hemorrhoids to get irritated.

Increasing fluid intake can also help ease constipation, and ultimately lead to less irritation to the affected area.

Non-steroidal anti-inflammatory drugs (NSAID's) can also be used to help alleviate symptoms. The most commonly used NSAID's are ibuprofen and naproxen, which can both help relieve pain and inflammation. If creams containing steroids are to be used, it is recommended that they not be used for more than fourteen days, as they can cause thinning of the skin.

If the condition requires it, a number of safe, office-based procedures may be performed to deal with people suffering from hemorrhoids. For those with minor hemorrhoids, the first line of treatment is typically rubber band litigation. This procedure involves applying elastic bands onto an internal hemorrhoid. The objective is to cut off the blood supply to the blood vessel in question. Once the blood supply has been cut off, the hemorrhoid begins to wither, and generally falls off within five to seven days. This method has been shown to be around eighty-five percent effective.

Sclerotherapy is another safe, office-based procedure that can be used to treat hemorrhoids. It involves an injection in order to make the vein shrink. The hemorrhoid will eventually shrivel up once the vein wall collapses. This has about a seventy percent success rate.

If other treatments fail, cauterization (the burning off of specific tissue) has proven to be somewhat effective for treating hemorrhoids. There are several types of cauterization methods, ranging from electrocautery, infrared radiation, laser surgery, or cryosurgery. Infrared cauterization is generally only considered an option for those with minor cases.

Chapter 4: Surgical Treatments

If conservative management of the hemorrhoid fails, and the situation is severe enough to require it, there are a number of surgical procedures that can be done to help treat the affected area. It is important to emphasize, however, that as is common with many surgeries, there are hazardous side effects to consider. The nerves that supply the bladder are very close to the rectum, and because of this, there is a chance that any surgery in that area will result in bleeding, infection, a narrowing of the anal canal, and a lack of ability to urinate easily. Also present is a very small risk of fecal incontinence, which is a loss of control over bowel functions, particularly of liquid. Because of these harmful side effects (which often times turn out to be worse than the hemorrhoid itself), people should consider any surgery carefully before deciding to go ahead with it.

The first type of hemorrhoid surgery is called excisional hemorrhoidectomy, and is used only in the most extreme cases. Most people experience a considerable amount of postoperative pain, and generally need a full two to four weeks for recovery. However, in people with severe hemorrhoids, there is greater potential for long-term benefit compared to the non-surgical procedure of rubber band litigation. For those that suffer from a clotted external hemorrhoid, it is usually the recommended treatment from doctors.

An alternative to the intrusive hemorrhoidectomy procedure is the minimally invasive, doppler-guided transanal hemorrhoidal dearterialization, which involves locating arterial blood inflow through the use of an ultrasound doppler. The tissue is then stitched back up and the arteries are "tied off." Though this procedure has a slightly higher recurrence rate, it has far fewer complications than the hemorrhoidectomy.

For people that suffer from less severe forms of hemorrhoids, a procedure called stapled hemorrhoidectomy, is typically recommended. It involves removing a large amount of the especially enlarged hemorrhoidal tissue, and then following that up with repositioning the remaining hemorrhoidal tissue back to its default position. While there is a far greater likelihood of having symptomatic hemorrhoids return compared with a normal hemorrhoidectomy, since the hemorrhoid is not completely removed, the stapling procedure is much less painful and is usually accompanied by a much faster healing time.

Chapter 5: Natural Remedies

If a hemorrhoid condition advances to the point where it becomes unsafe or intolerable, people should go seek medical attention, both to ease their pain and ensure that the inflamed area does not become a potential health risk. But to treat hemorrhoids in its' infancy, there are many natural, safe, and effective remedies that can be tried in the comfort of your own home.

Since it is believed that excessive straining during bowel movements are one of the causes of hemorrhoids, straining should be stopped altogether. Lifting heavy objects should be avoided, as should any other type of activity where excessive straining of the lower back and abdomen is involved. Prolonged periods of sitting (both on the toilet and off) should be avoided, as it puts unneeded stress on the lower abdominal area. If a sedentary lifestyle is unavoidable (because of office work, for example), be sure to take breaks frequently and walk around for a bit. Furthermore, to help make stool softer and easier to pass, you should drink plenty of fluids, and add some key items to your diet that are high in fiber, such as bran, apples, carrots, leafy greens, broccoli, pears, grains, and beans. Some other foods high in fiber include wheat spaghetti, cooked pearl barley, artichoke, almonds, brown rice, oatmeal, cooked peas, cooked sweet corn, and brussel sprouts.

In order to avoid irritating the area even more, try and keep your bottom clean at all times, wiping after bowel movements with an ultra-soft tissue paper, lightly wetted paper towels, or adult wipes. Utilizing baby wipes would even be a good choice, as some contain aloe, a soothing plant which is known for its' ability to heal abrasions and relieve pain in tender areas. You can even try applying aloe vera gel, witch hazel, or organic apple cider directly to the irritated area to help ease discomfort. Also, an icepack can help temporarily relieve pain and itching.

When preparing to bathe, prepare a sitz bath (a bath which consists of sitting in water up to your hips in order to treat the lower part of the body) by adding some epsom salts to the water and soaking for several minutes per day. This will help relieve the pain and itching in the affected area. This can also be achieved by soaking a cotton ball (or paper towel) with witch hazel or apple cider vinegar, and gently applying it to the hemorrhoids. Both witch hazel and apple cider vinegar are astringents (substances that will cause body tissues to shrink), and will therefore lower the amount of discomfort the inflamed vessels are causing. A salve (an ointment made to treat skin conditions) consisting of Horse Chestnut is often used to treat varicose veins, but has been known to be effective with hemorrhoids as well.

One of the worst things a patient with hemorrhoids can do is scratch the itchy area. Excessive scratching can cause even more bleeding, and can ultimately lead to the spread of infection. If it is necessary to relieve itching inside or around the anus, it is recommended that a tight fitting latex glove be worn to avoid scratching the hemorrhoids with your nails and making the condition worse. Witch hazel has been shown to be a good choice to help relieve itching and inflammation.

Along with the methods for reducing pain and itchiness mentioned above, people can also alter their diet and avoid foods such as soda, beer, coffee, and strong spices, all of which can contribute to irritating the anus as the stool passes through. If bleeding is present, people who suffer from hemorrhoids should raise their intake of Vitamin K, a vitamin involved in stopping bleeding. Foods such as green leafy vegetables and alfalfa have very high concentrations of Vitamin K. To further ease the pain and swelling associated with hemorrhoids, people can use a warm water enema (squirting liquid into the anal cavity will soothe the tissue and encourage bowel movements) or take an oatmeal bath throughout the day as needed.

Finally, applying an ice pack or cold compress will help with pain relief by shrinking the affected veins.

Consuming herbs such as red grape vine leaf, collinsonia root, buckthorn, parsley, stone root, white oak bark, and fargelin can help reduce pain and swelling. These items can be ingested orally in capsule form or taken in tea form. Before taking herbs in general, however, a medical professional should be consulted so as to avoid any harmful interaction with other drugs. Some other popular herbs for hemorrhoids include butcher's broom and horse chestnut. Drinking pomegranate juice has also been found to help relieve symptoms. Another popular remedy is Neem oil. After the affected area has been cleaned, add a few drops of Neem oil to each hemorrhoid once daily until they clear up.

Chapter 6: Prevention

As with any illness, quality prevention is always much easier and effective than treating the condition once it appears, and there are several easy steps you can take to help prevent hemorrhoids.

A balanced, healthy diet is always one of the best and easiest things you can do to prevent medical issues, but for preventing hemorrhoids specifically, a diet high in fiber is ideal. Dietary fiber, which is commonly referred to as roughage or bulk, consists of the parts of plant foods that the human body can't digest or absorb. Unlike fats, proteins, or carbohydrates, which our bodies break down and digest, fiber traverses the digestive tract largely intact, passing through the stomach, small intestine, and colon, and is passed naturally through bowel movements. Fiber is extremely helpful in preventing hemorrhoids because it greatly increases the weight and size of stool (by absorbing water and causing stool to be less liquidy), as well as softening it. Stool that is larger is released from the body more easily, which can help lower the chance of constipation and/or irregular stool, both of which are believed to cause hemorrhoids.

Plant-based foods that are rich in fiber are whole-wheat flour, wheat bran, nuts, beans, cauliflower, and potatoes. The Institute of Medicine recommends that men age fifty or younger should have daily fiber intake of thirty-eight grams, while men age fifty-one or older should consume thirty grams of fiber per day. For women age fifty or younger, the ideal fiber amount is twenty-five grams, and for women age fifty-one or older, that number lowers to twenty-one grams.

Hand in hand with a balanced, healthy diet is exercising regularly. Unnecessary body weight puts extra pressure on the lower abdominal area, which can lead to hemorrhoids. The closer you stay to recommended body weight (given height, age, etc.), the more likely you are to prevent hemorrhoids from occurring.

Not straining during bowel movements or during heavy lifting is another simple way to possibly prevent hemorrhoids. As previously mentioned, the onset of hemorrhoids may be due to increased intra-abdominal pressure. Any methods that will allow stool to pass easily through the digestive tract, such as high fiber intake, drinking lots of water (at least eight cups per day), exercising regularly, etc., will ultimately assist in preventing hemorrhoids.

Conclusion

I hope that you have enjoyed this book, and found the information presented in it both informative and helpful. Thankfully, hemorrhoids is a condition which very rarely turns into a life-threatening situation. However, if left untreated, the inflammation, itching, and bleeding associated with swollen veins in the rectal area can lead to very serious quality of life issues. Even though physicians are still not sure of what specifically causes the onset of hemorrhoids, readers are encouraged to maintain a healthy lifestyle and body weight by exercising frequently and consuming a variety of nutritional items (with a high fiber intake), consume in moderation potentially irritating items like beer, soda, and coffee, and avoid excessive straining and lower abdominal pressure caused by lifting heavy objects or prolonged periods of sitting.

Should the symptoms of hemorrhoids become noticeable, you are encouraged to try out any of the all-natural methods for relief or to seek medical advice. It is important to keep in mind, however, that should the condition become severe, a surgical procedure may become necessary. Therefore, do not hesitate to seek specialized medical attention if the situation demands it.

Again, thanks for purchasing this book, and I wish you the best of luck in treating your hemorrhoid condition or continuing to live a hemorrhoid-free lifestyle. Just know that if you suffer from hemorrhoids, you are not alone, and that there is a supportive community out there willing and able to assist you in dealing with the physical discomfort hemorrhoids can cause.

Finally, if you discovered at least one thing that has helped you or that you think would be beneficial to someone else, be sure to take a few seconds to easily post a quick positive review. As an author, your positive feedback is desperately needed. Your highly valuable five star reviews are like a river of golden joy flowing through a sunny forest of mighty trees and beautiful flowers! *To do your good deed in making the world a better place by helping others with your valuable insight, just leave a nice review.*

Thanks and Best of Luck

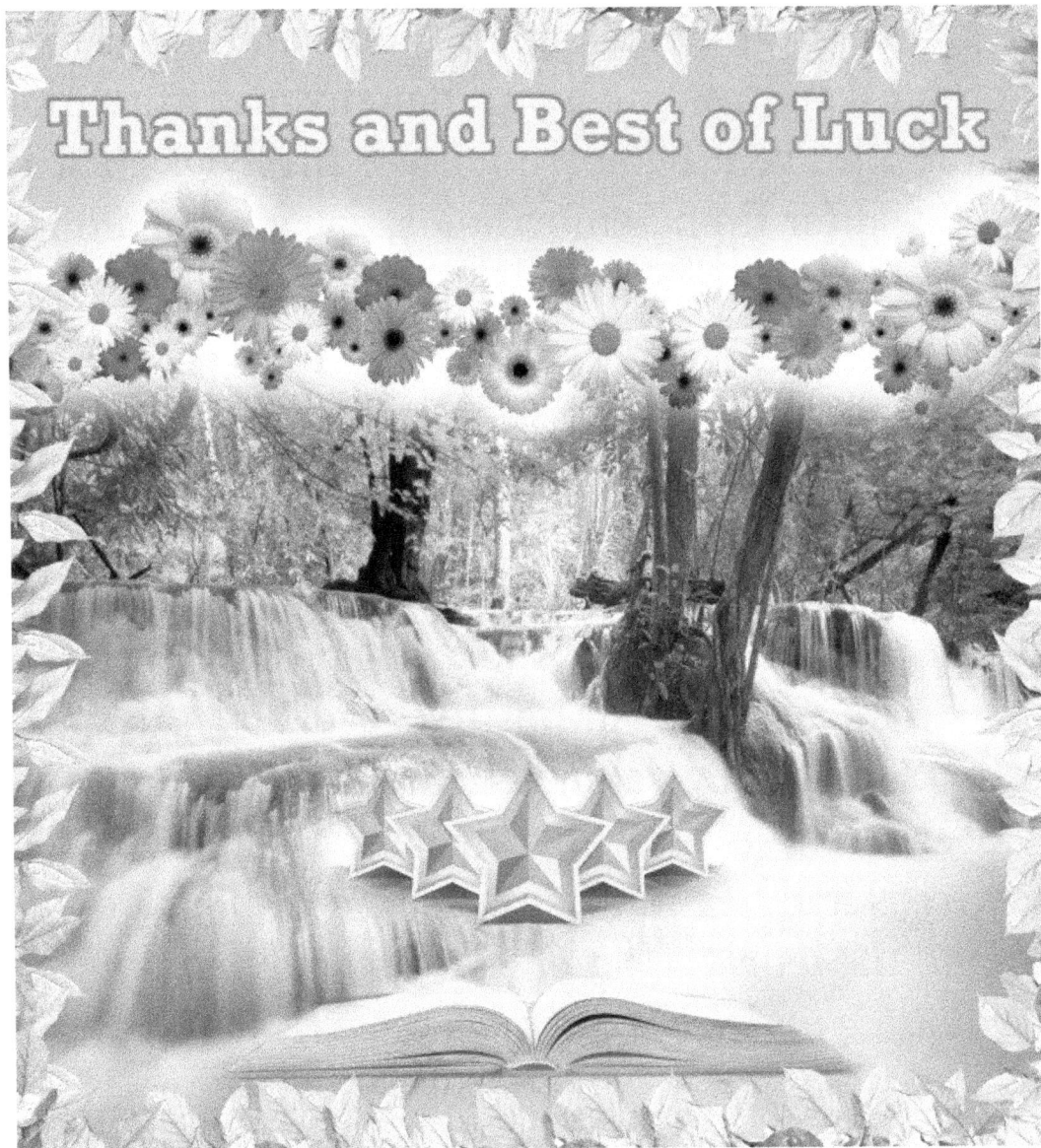

My Other Books and Audio Books

www.AcesEbooks.com

Health Books

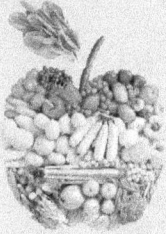

ULTIMATE HEALTH SECRETS

HEALTH

Strategies For Dieting, Eating Healthy, Exercising, Losing Weight, The Mediterranean Diet, Strength Training, And All About Vitamins, Minerals, And Supplements

Ace McCloud

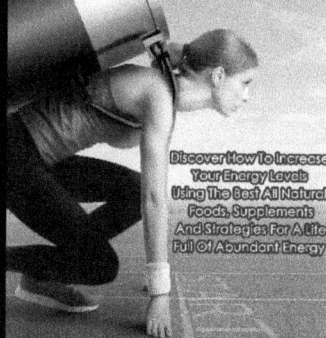

ENERGY
ULTIMATE ENERGY

Discover How To Increase Your Energy Levels Using The Best All Natural Foods, Supplements And Strategies For A Life Full Of Abundant Energy

Ace McCloud

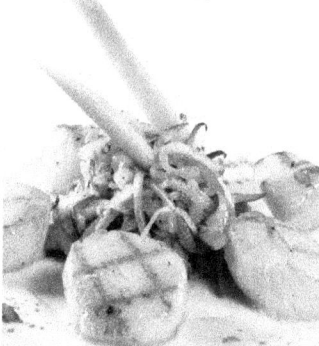

RECIPE BOOK

The Best Food Recipes That Are Delicious, Healthy, Great For Energy And Easy To Make

Ace McCloud

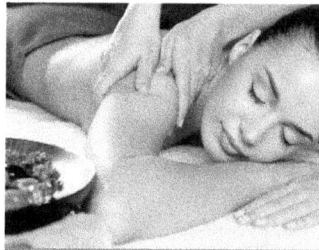

MASSAGE THERAPY

TRIGGER POINT THERAPY
ACUPRESSURE THERAPY
Learn The Best Techniques For Optimum Pain Relief And Relaxation

Ace McCloud

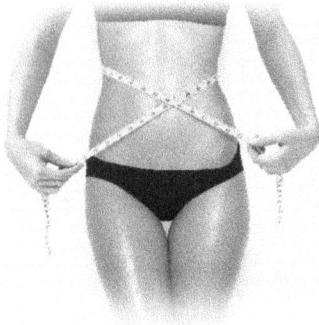

LOSE WEIGHT

THE TOP 100 BEST WAYS
TO LOSE WEIGHT QUICKLY AND HEALTHILY

Ace McCloud

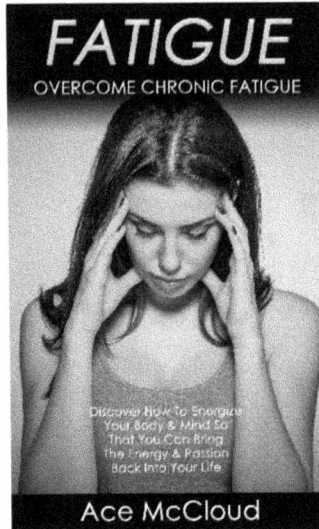

FATIGUE

OVERCOME CHRONIC FATIGUE

Discover How To Energize
Your Body & Mind So
That You Can Bring
The Energy & Passion
Back Into Your Life

Ace McCloud

Peak Performance Books

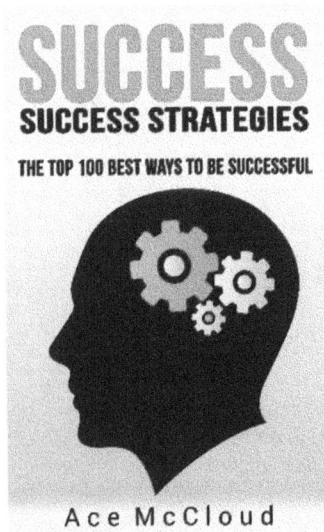

SUCCESS

SUCCESS STRATEGIES

THE TOP 100 BEST WAYS TO BE SUCCESSFUL

Ace McCloud

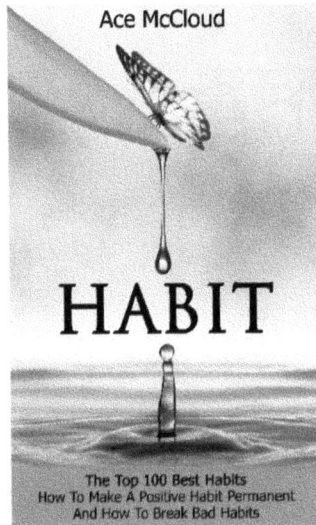

Ace McCloud

HABIT

The Top 100 Best Habits
How To Make A Positive Habit Permanent
And How To Break Bad Habits

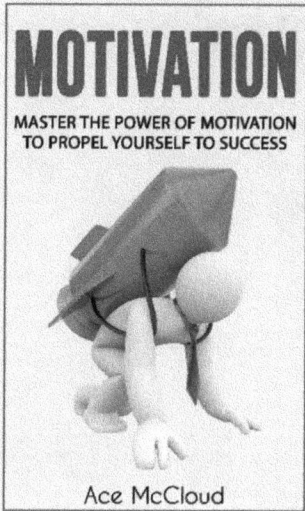

MOTIVATION

MASTER THE POWER OF MOTIVATION
TO PROPEL YOURSELF TO SUCCESS

Ace McCloud

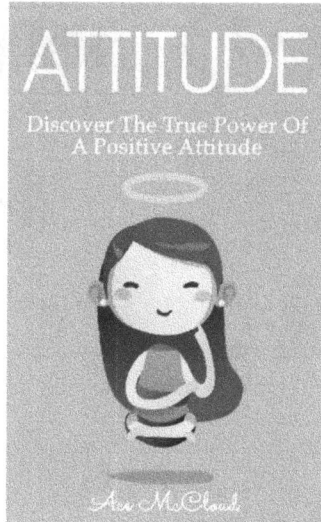

ATTITUDE

Discover The True Power Of
A Positive Attitude

Ace McCloud

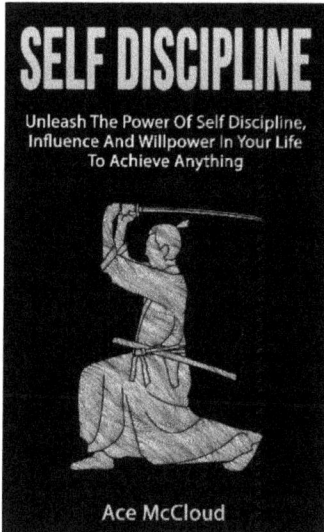

SELF DISCIPLINE

Unleash The Power Of Self Discipline,
Influence And Willpower In Your Life
To Achieve Anything

Ace McCloud

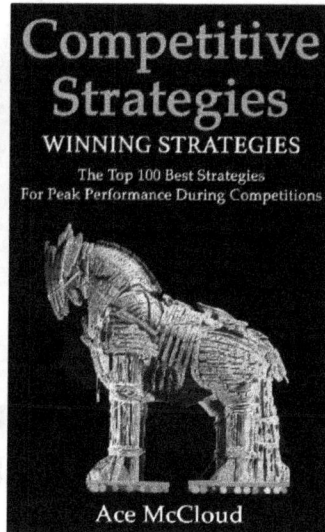

Competitive Strategies

WINNING STRATEGIES

The Top 100 Best Strategies
For Peak Performance During Competitions

Ace McCloud

Be sure to check out my audio books as well!

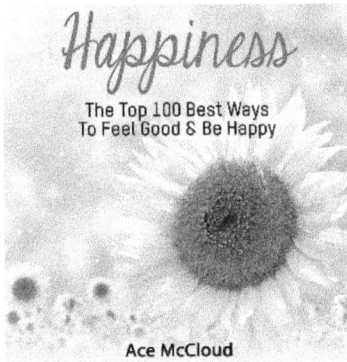

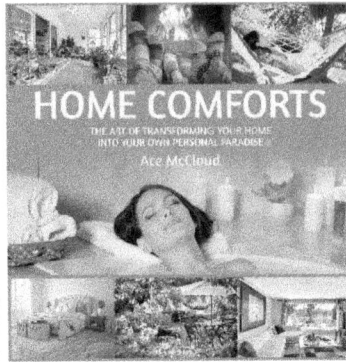

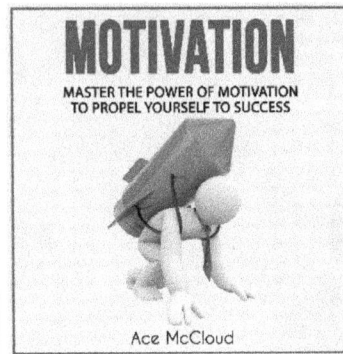

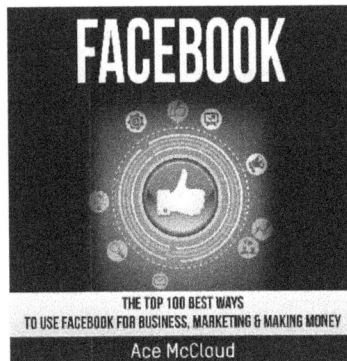

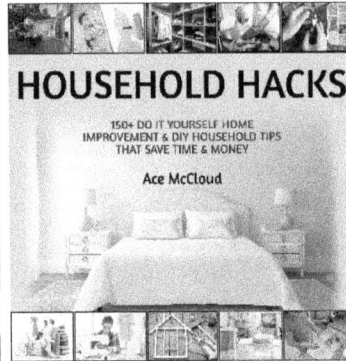

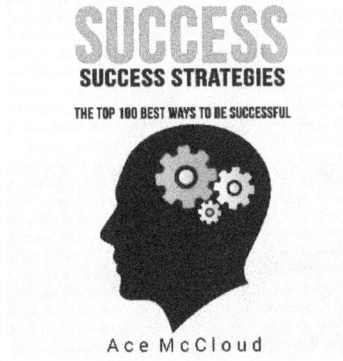

Check out my website at: www.AcesEbooks.com for a complete list of all of my books and high quality audio books. I enjoy bringing you the best knowledge in the world and wish you the best in using this information to make your journey through life better and more enjoyable! **Best of luck to you!**